Whole 30

Crockpot Cookbook

Quick and Easy
Whole 30 Crockpot Cookbook

Leslie Yothers

TABLE OF CONTENTS

WHAT IS THE CONCEPT OF WHOLE 30 AND THE WHOLE 30 CHALLENGE?

A Whole 30 diet refers to the 30-day marked diet that focuses on intake of whole food and elimination of alcohol, sugar, legumes, grains, dairy and soy from the meals. The Whole 30 diet is designed to put a restriction on unnecessary and irregular consumption of these items. The main aim of the program is to bring down the weight and stress levels by extracting energy from the right sources.

The list of food groups one is allowed to consume are:

- VEGETABLES

  Vegetables are an integral part of Whole 30 plan. The vegetables are low in calories and contain all types of nutrients. Consumption of vegetables also reduces the risk of diseases like diabetes and heart diseases. One must aim at including lots of vegetables in every meal. Green vegetables work the best.

- FRUITS

  One of the most common myths is that fruits contain hidden sugar which might affect one's diet. But here is the myth buster tip: Fruits contain natural sugar which is full of vitamins, fibers, and minerals. Fruits are included in the diet to bridge the gap of your sweet cravings. One must aim at consuming about 2 cups of fruits every day.

- FATS

  Fats don't increase your weight or make you fat! Fats, in turn, help you to absorb fat-soluble nutrients. They also keep you full that means, you will not feel hungry every now and then and your heart will be healthy too. Oils one must include in their plan are avocado oil, olive oil, coconut oil and canola oil. Other sources of healthy fats include olives, nuts, and avocado. One must avoid packaged food and items made up of hydrogenated oils in this diet program.

- PROTEINS

  Another important nutrient is protein that helps you build muscles, keep the skin clean and hairs shinier and healthy. One can find ample source of protein in eggs, yogurt nuts, meat, and seafood. One must aim at consuming proteins through whole meal foods only and should avoid sauces, protein shakes and bars.

The diet goes on for 30 days where participants have to abide by certain rules. They are advised not to measure their weight or calories in meanwhile. Once the diet program is completed, they are counseled to draw a personal list of food items, another list stating the health consequences as well as other useful information about the changes felt. The diet program has helped in curing various lifestyle-related conditions and diseases.

The diet has been distributed in certain phases which are mentioned as follows:

- STEP 1: SELECTING THE START DATE

  Planning plays an important role in the 30-day diet. Select a suitable start date while keeping every aspect in mind. Make sure to avoid any big, important or personal events or festivals in the month you are planning to perform this challenge. However, there is no one fixed date to perform the program, thus, whenever to decide to perform the challenge, make sure you perform it well without skipping a day.

- STEP 2: IMPOSING RESTRICTIONS

  This diet helps you awaken both mentally and physically. To achieve success in this program, one needs to impose certain restrictions and abide by the rules. The participant will have to cut down on certain food groups, replace the sources of energy and have a firm control over one's cravings. The book follows a list of foods to avoid and list of foods to consume on your diet journey.

- STEP 3: BELIEVING IN SELF

  Self-control and firm willpower is the key to success. One should believe that this diet is not hard and you can make through it. One should commit that they won't cheat their meals and will stick to the rules. The last but not the least, you can do this, you will do this!

- STEP 4: HIDING THE SCALES

Finally, you must hide the measuring scale. Yes, you read it right. The whole idea of following a Whole 30 diet is to transform into a healthier being, rather than focusing on weight loss like other diets. Though weight loss is one of the advantages of this diet, but still hiding the scales and not checking your weight for following 30 days will make you feel body positive.

Once you have prepared for all the four steps well, you are ready to embark upon the journey of changing your lifestyle with the Whole 30 program.

30 ADVANTAGES OF WHOLE 30 FOODS

- CONSISTENT ENERGY LEVELS: With changes in energy sources, you will notice a consistency in performing activities and working with faster speed than before.

- IMPROVED SLEEP SCHEDULES: With the elimination of sugars and intake of proteins or fats, your sleep will be for sound, longer and profound.

- BIDDING GOODBYE TO DIGESTIVE ISSUES: Digestive issues like indigestion, stomach aches etc. will take a back seat as the body will adapt to intake of more vegetables in this program.

- OPTIMISTIC APPROACH: You will feel better as the program will approach the end, waking up to more optimistic ideas every day.

- SWITCHING TO HEALTHIER OPTIONS: To boost in the fit lifestyle, the diet will include intake of a lot of vegetables. This will lead to better nutrition and healthier living.

- INCREASED WATER INTAKE: Since all the other drinks are restricted to this diet, your body's requirements will be met by water, which in turn will act as great measure.

- BEING HAPPY: With stability in blood sugar level, you will feel happy from inside. You will feel full and satisfied all day long.

- FOCUS AND DETERMINATION: Since the Whole 30 diet involves improving focus and alertness; you will find yourself more determined and getting clear ideas.

- SAVORING FOOD: Rather than gobbling and eating in excess, you will learn to appreciate the flavor and the nutrition you are gaining from every bite you eat. This will cut down the extra diet, thus, leading to weight loss.

- EMOTIONAL RELATIONSHIP WITH FOOD: With help of insulin management, the body will pass better signals about real hunger and appetite. This will help in avoiding unnecessary meals from day to day life. It will curb and remove the emotional attachment with food.

- PEACE OF MIND: The enhanced state of mind will help to remove anxiety and overthinking habits, thus, providing a calmness and peace to the brain. Since you will be happy, you will ultimately achieve the peace of mind too.

- EXPERIMENTING AND INVENTING: When you will indulge yourself in the Whole 30 plan, you will find yourself in the kitchen, experimenting with several ingredients and inventing your own personal dishes!

- NEW FAVORITES: With so many recipes to have around and by restricting the consumption of beans, grains, and dairy, you might notice a change in your taste or favorite dishes as well.

- KNOWING YOURSELF BETTER: By focusing on your body's demands and requirements for next 30 days, you will learn about your favorites, your dislikes, self-care, triggers, hunger periods etc.

- ORGANIZED LIFESTYLE: The most important concept behind the Whole 30 program is to organize your eating habits, leading to being better and organized in other sectors of life as well.

- MOTIVATION AND WILLPOWER: On this diet, you will find the motivation to continue it for the planned period of 30 days. You will feel the willpower rising within yourself with raised hormonal response and self-control over activities.

- INCREASED FERTILITY: Cutting down sugar will cut down the inflammation which is one of the biggest factors in lowering down the fertility in females. Thus, following this diet will be beneficial for the females who wish to increase their fertility rate naturally.

- CONTROLLING SUGAR: You will have a firm control over sugar intake and you will be able to curb your sugar demands after the end of the program, making a big difference.

- JOINT PAIN RELIEF: Removal of inflammation-causing foods reduces the inflammation around cushion pads of the knees, curing the issue of joint pain. Joint pain relief is usually experienced in adults, and following the whole 30 program will cure it.

- BALANCED HORMONES: With the right nutrients, your body will heal gradually, where you will experience lesser cravings and mood swings. You will be able to manage your insulin levels and glucose levels.

- CLEARER SKIN: Younger looking skin is just a diet away. You will feel a smooth and beautiful change in your skin with a natural glow after this program.

- LOSING WEIGHT: If the ultimate aim is losing weight, you can accomplish it with right types of meals. You might even develop some muscles with help of exercise.

- PRACTICAL NOTION OF FOOD: Food will not be the ultimate focus of your life; you will be able to look at the practical notion of it for developing a better version of yourself.

- ENHANCED WORKOUTS: Working out with consumption of right kind of food is nothing less than bliss to a healthy and fit life. Intake of fruits and vegetables along with the right type of exercise for your body will bring a major positive change in your life.

- MANAGING AND REMOVING DISEASES: The Whole 30 diet will reverse the symptoms of some diseases and cure other illnesses like asthma, diabetes etc. It also helps to fix and cure chronic diseases.

- SAYING NO TO BLOATING: As soon as the legumes and dairy products are gone, say bye to bloating too. Welcome flatter tummy!

- SHINIER HAIR, STRONGER NAILS: With enriched diet and right nutrients, you will get glossier and shinier hair. The problem of chipped nails will be solved with the growth of stronger nails.

- REDUCED OBSESSIONS ABOUT BEING OVERWEIGHT: Since one of the rules of the diet is that you cannot measure your weight, you will be focused on improving your way of leaving than losing weight or worrying about being overweight.

- INFLUENCING OTHERS: By sticking to the program schedule, not only you will develop an optimistic approach yourself, but also, you will be able to positively influence others preaching healthy lifestyle.

- ACCEPTANCE: By the end of the diet, you will able to accept the fact about your body, its image and will learn to love, care and celebrate the idea of being physically and mentally fit.

WHAT TO AVOID WHILE ON THE WHOLE 30 CHALLENGE?

While on a 30-day diet challenge, some foods are absolutely restricted. These food items are a complete no-no and are mentioned as follows:

- DAIRY

  Dairy products like cow milk, cheese, cream, yogurt, sour cream, and butter cannot be consumed while you are on a whole 30 challenge. However, there is an exception to the dairy rule that ghee can be consumed.

- ALCOHOL

  Alcohol cannot be used for drinking or cooking purposes while you choose the Whole 30 diet. This also means that you cannot intake any added flavors like vanilla extract etc.

- GRAINS

  Absolutely no rice, corn, quinoa, rye, wheat, sorghum, millet, buckwheat, amaranth, sprouted grains or bulgur for next 30 days!

- LEGUMES

  Another restricted component is legumes, meaning no beans, soy, tofu, miso, peas, chickpeas, peanuts or lentils for following 30 days. Cutting down legumes also helps to balance lots of issues well.

- JUNK

  Junk means something that you do not have to eat on this diet. No pizzas, pancakes, burgers etc. Try to emotionally cut off yourself from having junk to ensure success in this diet program.

- SULFITES AND MSG

  The participant should totally avoid consuming any type of processed food. Check the labels and avoid any items which include MSG, carrageenan or sulfites in it.

- SUGAR

  Sugar is present in various forms in various items. Cut down everything. Ignore any real or artificial intake in form of syrups, honey, stevia, agave etc. Check the label on everything and use items with no or minimal sugar level in them.

SIDE EFFECTS TO KNOW ABOUT

Whole 30 is not just a weight loss program, it is more of lifestyle treatment plan. With all the benefits involved, the diet comes up with side effects of its own which can sometimes weaken your willpower and motivation to continue the challenge. If you are looking to pick up this challenge, have a look at the list of side effects as well which you might experience in one of the thirty days.

- HUNGER

  Being new to any diet program is always hard. And one of the hardest things to do is curbing your hunger. Sudden outbreaks, cravings etc. will make you eat your favorite thing, which is restricted in the diet. That is why self-control is really important in this challenge.

- EUPHORIA

  While eating vegetables and organics, you will feel light headed and happy in the beginning. You will be able to see changes and become happy quickly. This is euphoria and it doesn't last long. After a short period of time, everything will subside and things will get back to reality.

- MOOD SWINGS

  Mood swings will take over you as soon as you choose the program and restrict yourself to consume some food items. In the initial days, you will feel cranky and irritated, which is quite normal. Don't worry, just take a bath or a massage and do things that make you calm and happy.

- DULLNESS AND SLUGGISHNESS

  You will notice a constant light headache, achy joints, and painfull body. Due to the restriction of carbs, you will feel low throughout the day. As the body will adapt to the refined energy source, it will slowly fade away sluggishness.

- GUILT

  Since the Whole 30 diet is really restrictive in nature, the participant might feel like cheating. Once they cheat, they are not able to come up off the guilt, which continues as a heavy side effect.

- STOMACH ISSUES

  Excess intake of anything is harmful. Since you suddenly switch to intake of excess vegetables, the level of fiber content in your body shoots up. Fiber may add to discomfort as it might lead to constipation or diarrhea. You might also experience stomach aches and bowels.

WHOLE 30 CROCKPOT APPETIZERS

CROCK POT MEATLOAF BITES

SERVING SIZE: 4 BITES
SERVINGS PER RECIPE: 12
CALORIES: 234
PREPARATION TIME: ABOUT 3 HOURS AND 12 MINUTES

INGREDIENTS:

Avocado oil- 1 tbsp.

Ground pork- 2 lbs.

Diced onion- 2 cups

Almond flour- ½ cup

Eggs- 2

Garlic powder- 1 tbsp.

Pepper flakes- 2 tsp

Dried oregano- 2 tsp

Fennel seeds- 2 tsp

Dried thyme- 2 tsp

Ground sage- 2 tsp

Sea salt- 1 tsp

Paprika- 1 tsp

Black pepper- 1 tsp

NUTRITION INFORMATION

Fat - 6 g

Fiber - 1 g

Carbohydrates - 17 g

Protein - 27 g

Cholesterol - 90 mg

INSTRUCTIONS:

1. Cook the onions in warm avocado oil till they are translucent.

2. Except for the pork, mix all the other ingredients in a large bowl. Stir until thoroughly mixed.

3. Now, add the onions and the pork to the mixture in the bowl.

4. Put all this mixture in the center of your crock pot.

5. Cover with a lid and cook for at least 3 hours on a low temperature setting. Make sure that the internal temperature of the meat is 150 degrees.

6. Let it rest for about 10 to 20 minutes then shift the meatloaf.

7. Refrigerate for 8 hours, then cut bite-size pieces.

8. Heat before serving.

ORANGE CARNITAS CRISPS

SERVING SIZE: 1 PLATE
SERVINGS PER RECIPE: 8
CALORIES: 300
PREPARATION TIME: 8 HOURS AND 15 MINUTES

INGREDIENTS:

Salt- 1 tsp

Pork shoulder- 3 lbs.

Oregano- 2 tsp

Pepper- ½ tsp

Chili powder- ½ tsp

Ground cumin- 1 tsp

Cinnamon stick- 1

Bay leaf- 1

Garlic- 6 cloves, minced

Onion- 1, chopped

Butter- 3 tbsp.

Oranges- 2, juiced

Lime- 1, juiced

NUTRITION INFORMATION

Fat-23 g

Fiber-0.2 g

Carbohydrates-2 g

Protein-19 g

Cholesterol-80 mg

INSTRUCTIONS:

1. Mix the pork with oregano, pepper, chili powder, salt, and cumin in a crock pot. Ensure that the meat is properly mixed with the spices.

2. Now, add bay leaf, garlic, onion, as well as cinnamon in the crockpot.

3. Add the orange juice and the lime juice and cover with the lid.

4. Start cooking on a low heat setting for about 7 to 8 hours.

5. After that, use a large fork to shred the cooked pork.

6. Put this shredded meat in a pan along with the butter to fry to make it crispy.

7. Serve with lime.

PORK TACOS

SERVING SIZE: 1 TACO
SERVINGS PER RECIPE: 8
CALORIES: 459
PREPARATION TIME: 8 HOURS AND 10 MINUTES

INGREDIENTS:

Bacon fat- 2 tbsp.

Pork shoulder- 2 ½ lbs, no bones

Black pepper- according to taste, freshly ground

Salt- according to taste

Orange- 1, juiced

Chicken broth- ¼ cup

Dried cumin- 2 tsp

Garlic- 4 cloves, chopped

Lime- 1, juiced

Onion- 1, chopped

Cayenne pepper- ½ tsp

Taco shells

Dried oregano- 2 tsp

NUTRITION INFORMATION

Fat-13 g

Fiber-4 g

Carbohydrates-43 g

Protein-39 g

Cholesterol-94 mg

INSTRUCTIONS:

1. Use paper towels to dry the pork shoulder. Coat it with sea salt and pepper.

2. Melt bacon fat in a large pan and cook the pork shoulder until it turns brown.

3. Now, fill your crock pot with the chicken broth. Put the cooked pork in the broth and add lime and orange juice.

4. Add cumin, garlic, cayenne pepper, onions, and oregano.

5. Cover with the lid and let it cook for about 7 to 8 hours on a low heat setting. Make sure that the meat is tender after cooking.

6. After cooking remove the onion pieces. Add additional salt according to your taste.

7. Carefully place the cooked meat in layers in a baking dish. Then, broil it in an oven for 2 to 6 minutes to get a crispy texture.

8. Put the meat with cilantro in taco shells. Serve.

SAUSAGE BELL PEPPER CUPS

SERVING SIZE: 1 PEPPER CUP
SERVINGS PER RECIPE: 5
CALORIES: 350
PREPARATION TIME: 6 HOURS AND 32 MINUTES

INGREDIENTS:

Bell peppers- 5

Ground sausage- 1 pound

Tomato paste- 1 can of 8 ounce

Cauliflower- ½ head, chopped

Garlic- ½ pod, minced

White onion- 1, small, diced

Dried thyme- 2 tsp

Dried oregano- 2 tsp

Fresh Basil- 1 bunch, minced

NUTRITION INFORMATION

Fat-14 g

Fiber-3 g

Carbohydrates-26 g

Protein-36 g

Cholesterol-98 mg

INSTRUCTIONS:

1. Cut the bell peppers at the top and scoop out the inside to give it a cup-like shape. You can use a knife to scoop out the seeds. Make sure you save the top portion.

2. In a large bowl, mix the chopped cauliflower, with basil, dried herbs, onion, and garlic. Use your hands to create a consistent mixture.

3. Brown the ground sausage in a large skillet.

4. Mix the cooked sausage with the cauliflower mixture and tomato paste.

5. Fill this mixture inside every bell pepper.

6. Place the filled peppers in your crock pot and cover them with their tops.

7. Cook this for about 5 to 6 hours on a low heat setting.

8. Take out and serve.

SLOW COOKER STYLE SPICY SWEET POTATO

SERVING SIZE: 1 BOWL
SERVINGS PER RECIPE: 10
CALORIES: 230
PREPARATION TIME: 12 HOURS AND 15 MINUTES

INGREDIENTS:

Onion- 1, diced

Ground beef- 2 lbs.

Tomatoes- 14 oz., minced

Tomato sauce- 14 oz.

Garlic- 1 clove, minced

Sweet potato- 1, large, diced after peeling

Beef stock- 3 cups

Salt- 2 tsp

Chili powder- 3 to 4 tbsp.

Black pepper- ½ tsp

Cilantro for garnishing

Oregano- ¼ tsp

NUTRITION INFORMATION

Fat-3 g

Fiber-12 g

Carbohydrates-45 g

Protein-12 g

Cholesterol-0 mg

INSTRUCTIONS:

1. . Keep the beef over medium heat and cook it properly till brown. This will melt the extra fat, which you can then easily remove.

2. Put this meat into your crockpot, and add the rest of the ingredients. Stir properly to combine all the ingredients.

3. Let it cook for about 7 to 8 hours on a slow heat setting. Then, increase the heat setting to high and cook for a further 2 to 4 hours.

4. Properly stir to shred and mix the meat in the mixture.

5. Garnish with cilantro and serve warm.

GARLIC CAULIFLOWER MASH

SERVING SIZE: 1 SMALL BOWL
SERVINGS PER RECIPE: 6
CALORIES: 66
PREPARATION TIME: 8 HOURS AND 16 MINUTES

INGREDIENTS:

Garlic- 6 cloves

Cauliflower- 1, large

Pepper and salt- according to taste

Dill- 1 package, fresh

Coconut milk

NUTRITION INFORMATION

Fat-4 g

Fiber-2 g

Carbohydrates-6 g

Protein-2 g

Cholesterol-10 mg

INSTRUCTIONS:

1. Get rid of the base and the exterior leaves of the cauliflower. Cut the florets of this cauliflower head and put it in a crock pot.

2. Add half the dill and the garlic to the crockpot.

3. Fill the crockpot with water until all the florets are submerged.

4. Cover the lid and let it cook for about 7 to 8 hours on a low temperature setting.

5. After cooking, carefully remove the cooked cauliflower as well as the garlic in a large bowl. Get rid of the dill in the pot.

6. Add pepper and salt to the bowl and mix coconut milk and the rest of the dill.

7. Finally, use a blender to pulse this mixture to a consistent texture.

8. Use as an appetizer whenever you need.

SLOW COOKED GREEN BEANS AND KALE

SERVING SIZE: 1 BOWL
SERVINGS PER RECIPE: 4
CALORIES: 254
PREPARATION TIME: 5 HOURS AND 12 MINUTES

INGREDIENTS:

Coconut milk- 1 can

Kale- 1, medium, chopped into big chunks

Chicken stock- 1 can

Green beans- 2 handfuls, ends trimmed

Curry powder- 1 tbsp.

NUTRITION INFORMATION

Fat-8 g

Fiber-9 g

Carbohydrates-31 g

Protein-14 g

Cholesterol-0 mg

INSTRUCTIONS:

1. Add chicken stock and coconut milk to your crock pot.

2. Add the curry powder and mix.

3. Add the green beans and stir properly.

4. Add the kale and coat it with the thick liquid.

5. Close and cook for about 3 to 5 hours on a low heat setting.

6. Remove the excess liquid and serve.

APPLE AND CINNAMON SAUCE

SERVING SIZE: ¾ CUP
SERVINGS PER RECIPE: 10
CALORIES: 89
PREPARATION TIME: 8 HOURS AND 5 MINUTES

INGREDIENTS:

Sweet apples- 6, cored and peeled

Water- 1 tbsp.

Granny Smith apple- 6, cored and peeled

Cinnamon- 1 tsp

Nutmeg- 1 pinch

NUTRITION INFORMATION

Fat-0 g

Fiber-4 g

Carbohydrates-23 g

Protein-0 g

Cholesterol-0 mg

INSTRUCTIONS:

1. Put all the ingredients in your crock pot.

2. Cover with the lid and let it cook for about 7 to 8 hours on a low heat setting.

3. This can be served warm after cooking or chilled for later.

SLOW COOKER SALMON FRITTATA BITES

SERVING SIZE: 1 PIECE
SERVINGS PER RECIPE: 6
CALORIES: 133
PREPARATION TIME: 2 HOURS AND 30 MINUTES

INGREDIENTS:

Eggs- 10

Salmon fillets- 1 ½ lb.

Small onion- ½

Dill- 1 tbsp., chopped

Cooking oil- 2 tbsp.

Chives- 1 tsp

Capers- 1 tbsp., chopped

Pepper and salt- according to taste

NUTRITION INFORMATION

Fat-6 g

Fiber-0 g

Carbohydrates-2 g

Protein-17 g

Cholesterol-166 mg

INSTRUCTIONS:

1. Cut the salmon fillets into small pieces.

2. Coat each side with pepper and salt.

3. Line a crock pot with a quality parchment paper. Now place the fillets in the crock pot and let it cook for about 2 hours on a high heat setting.

4. Take out the cooked pieces and place them on a large baking sheet greased with butter.

5. To a large bowl add capers, dill, eggs, chives, and pepper with salt. Mix thoroughly.

6. Now, pour this mixture all over the fish pieces.

7. Bake in the oven for 20 to 30 minutes.

8. Take out the baking sheet and let it cool for at least 8 to 10 minutes.

9. Serve warm.

TOMATO ONION EGG FRITTATA

SERVING SIZE: 1 PIECE
SERVINGS PER RECIPE: 4
CALORIES: 146
PREPARATION TIME: 2 HOURS AND 6 MINUTES

INGREDIENTS:

Eggs- 6

Mushrooms- 4 oz., sliced

Italian seasoning- 2 tsp

Spinach- ¼ cup, chopped

Green onions- 2, sliced

Butter- 1 tsp, clarified

Cherry tomatoes- ¼ cup, sliced

NUTRITION INFORMATION

Fat-8 g

Fiber-1 g

Carbohydrates-7 g

Protein-10 g

Cholesterol-189 mg

INSTRUCTIONS:

1. Use cooking spray to properly grease the interior of the crock pot.

2. Sauté all the vegetables in warm butter in a large pan. Make sure you stop cooking as soon as the vegetables are tender.

3. Now, put all these vegetables into your crock pot.

4. Use a large bowl to mix the eggs with seasoning.

5. Add this mixture to the crock pot too.

6. Cover and cook on a high temperature setting for about 2 hours. Make sure you don't open the lid during this time.

7. Remove and cut four pieces to serve. Use your favorite toppings such as green onion pieces, lime juice, and cilantro to garnish.

WHOLE 30 CROCKPOT POULTRY RECIPES

SLOW COOKER CASHEWS AND CHICKEN THIGHS

SERVING SIZE: 1 PLATE
SERVINGS PER RECIPE: 6
CALORIES: 322
PREPARATION TIME: 3 HOURS AND 20 MINUTES

INGREDIENTS:

Tapioca flour- ¼ cup

Chicken thighs- 2 lbs., cut into pieces, skin and bones removed

Black pepper- ½ tsp

Onions- 2, green, chopped

Coconut oil- 2 tbsp.

Tomato paste- 2 tbsp., organic

Garlic- 3 cloves, minced

Ginger- 1/2, freshly minced

Palm sugar- 1 tbsp.

Apple cider vinegar- 2 tbsp.

Sesame oil- 1 tbsp.

Cashews- ½ cup

Pepper flakes- 1 pinch

Sea salt- ½ tsp

NUTRITION INFORMATION

Fat-7 g

Fiber-4 g

Carbohydrates-36 g

Protein-29 g

Cholesterol-65 mg

INSTRUCTIONS:

1. Take a large Ziploc bag mix the tapioca flour with black pepper. Add the chicken pieces and properly coat with the mixture.

2. Take a medium-sized pan and warm the coconut oil. Add the coated chicken pieces to the pan and cook by stirring for about 1 to 2 minutes. Keep the heat on a medium setting during this time.

3. Now, you can mix the rest of the available ingredients in a large enough bowl.

4. Stir the chicken with the prepared mixture and put it in a crock pot.

5. Cover and let it cook for about 3 hours on a low heat setting. Keep the lid closed and do not open during this cooking time. You can open after 2 and ½ hours during this three-hour period.

6. Serve with additional green onion pieces.

TANGY SLOW COOKER CHICKEN WITH GARLIC AND THYME

SERVING SIZE: 1 PLATE
SERVINGS PER RECIPE: 6
CALORIES: 167
PREPARATION TIME: 10 HOURS AND 20 MINUTES

INGREDIENTS:

Lemon juice- ¼ cup, freshly squeezed

Chicken- 4 lbs, whole

Bay leaves- 3

Thyme- 5 sprigs, fresh

Black pepper- ¼ tsp

Garlic- 5 cloves, peeled

Salt- 1 tsp

NUTRITION INFORMATION

Fat-5 g

Fiber-0.2 g

Carbohydrates-0.9 g

Protein-27 g

Cholesterol-73 mg

INSTRUCTIONS:

1. Use cool water to properly rinse your chicken.

2. Put the chicken into your crock pot.

3. Squeeze the lemon juice all over the chicken in the crock pot. Also, add thyme, pepper, and salt.

4. Surround the chicken with bay leaves and garlic cloves.

5. Set the crock pot for a low heat cooking for about 8 to 10 hours.

6. Check that if the meat is easily leaving the bone.

7. Serve with vegetables.

CILANTRO LIME CHICKEN DRUMSTICKS

SERVING SIZE: 3 DRUMSTICKS
SERVINGS PER RECIPE: 6
CALORIES: 225
PREPARATION TIME: 2 HOURS AND 46 MINUTES

INGREDIENTS:

Chicken drumsticks- 4 lbs.
Lime- 2, small
Salt- 1 tsp
Cilantro- ¼ cup, chopped
Pepper- 1/2 tsp
Garlic- ½ tbsp., minced

NUTRITION INFORMATION

Fat-3 g
Fiber-4 g
Carbohydrates-19 g
Protein-29 g
Cholesterol-70 mg

INSTRUCTIONS:

1. Squeeze the limes into the crock pot. Add cilantro, garlic, pepper and salt. Mix properly.

2. Add the chicken drumsticks and properly mix the spices to coat the chicken.

3. Cover with the lid and let it cook for about 2 to 3 hours on a high temperature setting. Don't open the lid of the crock pot.

4. After cooking in the crock pot. Bake in a preheated oven at 500 degrees for at least 8 to 10 minutes.

5. Use the juices collected in the crock pot at the time of serving.

ZUCCHINI KALE CHICKEN SOUP

SERVING SIZE: 1 BOWL
SERVINGS PER RECIPE: 6
CALORIES: 169
PREPARATION TIME: 6 HOURS AND 35 MINUTES

INGREDIENTS:

Chicken breasts- 2 lbs., skinless and boneless

Yellow onion- 1, chopped

Tomato paste- 1 can of 15 oz.

Garlic powder- 1 tsp

Cumin- 1 tsp

Chili powder- ½ tsp, mild

Chicken broth- 32 oz. package, low-sodium

Kosher salt- 3 tsp

Zucchini- 3, medium, chopped

Water- 4 cups

Kale- 3 cups, chopped

Cherry tomatoes- 1 pint, divided

Lime juice- 2

NUTRITION INFORMATION

Fat-2 g

Fiber-4 g

Carbohydrates-20 g

Protein-17 g

Cholesterol-35 mg

INSTRUCTIONS:

1. To your crock pot add tomato paste, chicken, onion, garlic powder, cumin, water, chicken broth, chili powder and salt.

2. Close the lid and let this mixture cook for about 5 to 6 hours on a low heat setting. Make sure you check the chicken with the help of a fork.

3. Take out the cooked chicken and shred properly. Then, put it back in the crock pot and add the kale and zucchini.

4. Cool for extra 32 minutes to get tender veggies.

5. Mix properly after adding lime juice and use your favorite veggies as toppings.

CROCK POT BUTTER CHICKEN THIGHS

SERVING SIZE: 1 PLATE
SERVINGS PER RECIPE: 6
CALORIES: 189
PREPARATION TIME: 5 HOURS AND 32 MINUTES

INGREDIENTS:

Garlic- 4 cloves, crushed

Coconut oil- 1 tbsp.

Coconut milk- 1 ¾ cups

Onion- 1, diced

Tapioca flour- 2 tbsp.

Tomato paste- ¾ cup

Curry powder- 1 tsp

Indian gram masala- 2 tsp

Chili powder- ½ tsp

Ginger powder- ½ tsp

Pepper and salt- according to taste

Coriander- fresh

Chicken thighs- 1.25 kg, pieces

NUTRITION INFORMATION

Fat-6 g

Fiber-2 g

Carbohydrates-19 g

Protein-14 g

Cholesterol-70 mg

INSTRUCTIONS:

1. Use a saucepan to warm coconut oil at medium temperature heat.

2. Add garlic and onion and stir cook for about 2 to 3 minutes, to get a translucent texture of onion slices.

3. Include tomato paste, coconut milk, garam masala, tapioca flour, chili powder, ginger powder, and curry powder. Stir cook for a further 1 minute to get a thick consistency. Finally, add pepper and salt.

4. Now put the chicken thigh pieces in the crock pot. Mix properly with the prepared sauce.

5. Cover with the lid and let it cook for about 5 to 6 hours on a low temperature setting.

6. Garnish with coriander at the time of serving.

HATCH CHILI TOMATILLOS CHICKEN

SERVING SIZE: 1 PLATE
SERVINGS PER RECIPE: 6
CALORIES: 112
PREPARATION TIME: 5 HOURS AND 25 MINUTES

INGREDIENTS:

Cumin- 2 tsp

Chicken thighs- 3 lbs., skinless and boneless

Coriander- 1 tsp, ground

Sea salt- 1 ½ tsp

Tomatillos- 4, husked and diced

Black pepper- 1 tsp

Garlic- 3 cloves, finely chopped

Hatch green chili- ½ lb., diced

Onion- 1, medium, diced

Lime and cilantro- to garnish

NUTRITION INFORMATION

Fat-2 g

Fiber-3 g

Carbohydrates-14 g

Protein-9 g

Cholesterol-15 mg

INSTRUCTIONS:

1. Place the chicken thigh pieces at the bottom of your crock pot.

2. Add coriander, black pepper and cumin. Make sure you properly toss every chicken piece with this seasoning.

3. Also add the garlic, green chilies, tomatillos and the onions to the crock pot.

4. Cook this covered with the lid for about 5 to 6 hours on a low temperature setting.

5. After cooking, use a fork to shred the cooked meat.

BALSAMIC PEACH AND BASIL CHICKEN

SERVING SIZE: 1 PLATE
SERVINGS PER RECIPE: 6
CALORIES: 202
PREPARATION TIME: 6 HOURS AND 15 MINUTES

INGREDIENTS:

White onion- 1, large, sliced

Chicken breasts- 1 lb., skin and bone removed

Salt- 2 tsp

Balsamic vinegar- ¼ cup

Peaches- 6, sliced

Garlic powder- 1 tsp

Basil leaves- ¼ cup, sliced

NUTRITION INFORMATION

Fat-3 g

Fiber-4 g

Carbohydrates-22 g

Protein-20 g

Cholesterol-71 mg

INSTRUCTIONS:

1. Carefully make a layer of onion slices in your crock pot. Pour the vinegar and add the garlic powder and salt to this layer. Now, mix the slices of peaches, but keep two peaches for after.

2. Add the chicken pieces to the crock pot. Properly coat with the mixture already available in the pot.

3. Set the crock pot on a low heat setting and cook for about 5 to 6 hours.

4. After cooking, take out the chicken and shred it with the help of a fork.

5. Put the shredded chicken back in the crock pot and add more vinegar and salt if required. Stir to mix, add the rest of the sliced peaches and basil.

6. Serve.

CHICKEN BREASTS WITH SALSA

SERVING SIZE: 1 PLATE
SERVINGS PER RECIPE: 6
CALORIES: 177
PREPARATION TIME: 6 HOURS AND 15 MINUTES

INGREDIENTS:

Onions- 2, medium, sliced

Chicken breasts- 2 lbs., skin and bone removed

Salsa- 1 can, no sugar

Bell pepper- 2 medium, sliced

Lime juice- 1

Salt- ½ tsp

NUTRITION INFORMATION

Fat-4 g

Fiber-2 g

Carbohydrates-7 g

Protein-27 g

Cholesterol-72 mg

INSTRUCTIONS:

1. Mix the peppers, onions, chicken, salt and salsa in your crock pot.

2. Cover with the lid and let it cook for about 5 to 6 hours on a low heat setting.

3. Remove the lid and take out the cooked chicken on to a board. Use forks to shred the chicken.

4. Add the shredded chicken to the mixture in the crock pot and enhance the tangy flavor with lime juice and serve.

PULLED CHICKEN WITH CRISP APPLES

SERVING SIZE: 1 PLATE
SERVINGS PER RECIPE: 6
CALORIES: 312
PREPARATION TIME: 6 HOURS AND 10 MINUTES

INGREDIENTS:

Onion- 1, medium, sliced

Crisp apples- 2, sweet, chopped

Kosher salt- 1 tsp

Apple cider- ¾ cup, no sweetness, divided

Garlic powder- 1 tsp, granulated

Chicken breasts- 2 lbs., skin and bone removed

NUTRITION INFORMATION

Fat-5 g

Fiber-0.3 g

Carbohydrates-20 g

Protein-46 g

Cholesterol-122 mg

INSTRUCTIONS:

1. In your crock pot, add a layer of onions and apple slices. Add a little salt and toss properly.

2. Use garlic powder and salt to thoroughly coat the chicken.

3. Put this chicken in the crock pot with the onion and apple slices. Add half a cup of the apple cider.

4. Now, you can cover the pot and set it on a low temperature setting to cook for about 5 to 6 hours.

5. Take out the cooked chicken from the pot and shred it using a large fork. Add the shredded meat to the pot again with more apple cider. Mix and adjust salt and cider according to your taste.

CROCK POT CHICKEN PIE

SERVING SIZE: 1 PIE SLICE
SERVINGS PER RECIPE: 6
CALORIES: 480
PREPARATION TIME: 8 HOURS AND 30 MINUTES

INGREDIENTS:

Carrot- 3 cups, chopped
Yellow onion- 2 cups, chopped
Celery- 2 cups, chopped
Chicken stock- 32 oz.
Kosher salt- 1 tsp
Chicken breast- 2 lbs., skin and bone removed
Bay leaf- 1
Coconut milk- ¾ cup

NUTRITION INFORMATION

Fat-24 g
Fiber-1 g
Carbohydrates-33 g
Protein-30 g
Cholesterol-93 mg

INSTRUCTIONS:

1. Stir to mix the carrot, onion chicken stock, salt, and celery in your crock pot. Now, add the bay leaf and chicken breasts.

2. Mix and cover the pot with the lid and cook for about 7 to 8 hours on a low temperature setting.

3. Take out the chicken and use a large fork to shred it. Put the shredded chicken into the pot again and add coconut milk. Add more salt if required.

4. Serve warm.

PULLED CHICKEN WITH TANGY HERB SAUCE

SERVING SIZE: 1 PLATE
SERVINGS PER RECIPE: 6
CALORIES: 247
PREPARATION TIME: 6 HOURS AND 10 MINUTES

INGREDIENTS:

Lemon juice- 1/3 cup, freshly squeezed
Garlic- 4 cloves, grated
Dijon mustard- 1 tsp
Olive oil- 1/3 cup
Kosher salt- ½ tsp
Italian seasoning- 1 tsp
Chicken breasts- 2 lbs., skin and bone removed

NUTRITION INFORMATION

Fat-4 g
Fiber-7 g
Carbohydrates-27 g
Protein-24 g
Cholesterol-46 mg

INSTRUCTIONS:

1. Use a medium-sized bowl to create your tangy sauce. Mix lemon juice, garlic, salt and mustard. Whisk in olive oil and add Italian seasoning and stir until every ingredient blends together.

2. Now your sauce is ready, you can add it to the chicken in your crock pot.

3. Cook with a covered lid for about 5 to 6 hours on a low heat setting.

4. Remove the chicken on a board and shred it properly. Make sure you use a fork to do so. Then, put this chicken back into the pot and mix properly with the sauce.

5. Serve.

HOT CHICKEN WITH SWEET POTATO

SERVING SIZE: 1 PLATE
SERVINGS PER RECIPE: 8
CALORIES: 234
PREPARATION TIME: 6 HOURS AND 15 MINUTES

INGREDIENTS:

Chicken breasts- 1 ½ lbs., bone and skin removed
Coconut oil- 1 ½ tbsp.
Hot sauce- ¾ cup, red sauce with a few ingredients
Sweet potatoes- 4, small

NUTRITION INFORMATION

Fat-4 g
Fiber-4 g
Carbohydrates-30 g
Protein-18 g
Cholesterol-32 mg

INSTRUCTIONS:

1. Take a medium-sized bowl to mix 1 tbsp. of oil with hot sauce.

2. Use the rest of the oil to coat the sweet potatoes with skin-on.

3. Now, put the chicken breasts in your crock pot. Use the prepared sauce to coat the chicken all over.

4. Place the sweet potatoes over the chicken pieces in the pot.

5. Seal the lid and let it cook for about 5 to 6 hours on a low temperature setting. Make sure that chicken and potatoes are tender.

6. Take out the chicken, shred it and put it back to mix with the sauce.

7. Take out the potatoes and slice them.

8. Serve chicken with sweet potato slices.

ITALIAN CHICKEN STEW WITH RED POTATOES

SERVING SIZE: 1 BOWL
SERVINGS PER RECIPE: 8
CALORIES: 202
PREPARATION TIME: 6 HOURS AND 15 MINUTES

INGREDIENTS:

Celery- 1 cup, chopped

Onion- 1 cup, chopped

Carrots- 1 cup, chopped

Chicken breasts- 1 lb., skinless and boneless

Red potatoes- 1 cup, chopped

Tomato paste- 1 can of 6 oz.

Roasted tomato- 1 can of 15 oz.

Italian seasoning- 1 tsp, dried

Chicken stock- 32 oz.

Garlic powder- 1 tsp, granulated

Kosher salt- ½ tsp

Olive oil- 2 tbsp.

Balsamic vinegar- 1 tbsp.

NUTRITION INFORMATION

Fat-3 g

Fiber-4 g

Carbohydrates-22 g

Protein-20 g

Cholesterol-71 mg

INSTRUCTIONS:

1. Prepare your crock pot by adding celery, carrots, tomato, onion, tomato paste, garlic and chicken to it. Also, add olive oil as well as balsamic vinegar.

2. Cook by covered with the lid for about 5 to 6 hours on a low temperature setting. This will tenderize the chicken and the vegetables.

3. Add a little water if desired to get the required consistency.

4. Take out the chicken breasts to shred them using a large fork. Stir back in the pot and add extra salt if needed.

5. Drizzle with olive oil before serving.

WHOLE 30 CROCKPOT SEAFOOD RECIPES

TILAPIA STEW WITH COCONUT MILK

SERVING SIZE: 1 BOWL
SERVINGS PER RECIPE: 6
CALORIES: 260 KCAL
PREPARATION TIME: 50 MINUTES

INGREDIENTS:

Tilapia- 2 lbs., fillets, cut into pieces

Lime juice- 4 tbsp.

Paprika- 1 ½ tbsp.

Ground cumin- 1 ½ tbsp.

Salt- 1 ½ tsp

Garlic- 2 ½ tsp, minced

Pepper- 1 ½ tsp

Onion- 1, large, chopped

Olive oil- 1 tbsp.

Bell peppers- 3, large, sliced

Cilantro- 1 bunch, fresh

Coconut milk- 14 oz.

NUTRITION INFORMATION

Fat-9 g

Fiber-2 g

Carbohydrates-11 g

Protein-31 g

Cholesterol-75 mg

INSTRUCTIONS:

1. Take a large bowl to mix cumin, lime juice, garlic, pepper, paprika and salt.

2. Coat every tilapia piece with this mixture.

3. Leave the coated fish fillets in the refrigerator to marinate. This will require at least 20 to 30 minutes.

4. Now, put olive oil in your crock pot and add onions. Keep the heat high and use a spoon to cook the onions for at least 2 to 3 minutes.

5. Now, add the tilapia, tomatoes and pepper slices to the crock pot too.

6. Add coconut milk and cook for about 40 to 50 minutes on a low temperature setting. Make sure you keep stirring from time to time.

7. Then, add cilantro and mix properly.

8. Serve warm.

AVOCADO LEEK GARLIC SALMON SOUP

SERVING SIZE: 1 BOWL
SERVINGS PER RECIPE: 4
CALORIES: 119
PREPARATION TIME: 40 MINUTES

INGREDIENTS:

Leeks- 4, washed and trimmed

Avocado oil- 2 tbsp.

Chicken broth- 6 cups

Garlic- 3 cloves, minced

Thyme leaves, 2 tsp, dried leaves

Coconut milk- 1 ¾ cup

Salmon- 1 lb., cut into pieces

Pepper and salt- according to taste

NUTRITION INFORMATION

Fat-3 g

Fiber-3 g

Carbohydrates-11 g

Protein-14 g

Cholesterol-35 mg

INSTRUCTIONS:

1. Use a saucepan to cook the leeks in the warmed avocado oil. Make sure that the leeks get only slightly soft.

2. Now, add the chicken stock, thyme and cooked leeks to your crock pot. Mild cook for about 10 to 15 minutes on a high setting.

3. Add pepper and salt if desired.

4. Put the salmon pieces along with the coconut milk and cook for another 10 minutes on the high setting.

5. Serve warm.

CILANTRO LEMON SHRIMP CURRY

SERVING SIZE: 1 PLATE
SERVINGS PER RECIPE: 4
CALORIES: 243
PREPARATION TIME: 4 HOURS AND 35 MINUTES

INGREDIENTS:

Coconut milk- 30 oz.

Shrimp- 1 lb.

Lemon and garlic- 2 ½ tsp, for seasoning

Water- 15 oz.

Cilantro- ¼ cup

Curry paste- 2 tbsp.

NUTRITION INFORMATION

Fat-7 g

Fiber-2 g

Carbohydrates-12 g

Protein-28 g

Cholesterol-190 mg

INSTRUCTIONS:

1. Put the seasoning, coconut milk, curry paste, water and cilantro in the crock pot. Make sure you mix everything well.

2. Start cooking on a low heat temperature for about 4 hours.

3. Add the shrimp and let it cook for another 20 to 30 minutes. Check the shrimp and take them out.

4. Use plenty of cilantro for garnishing.

TANGY SALMON WITH FRESH DILL

SERVING SIZE: 1 PLATE
SERVINGS PER RECIPE: 4
CALORIES: 210
PREPARATION TIME: 2 HOURS AND 10 MINUTES

INGREDIENTS:

Fresh dill- 1 handful

Salmon- 2 lb.

Lemon- 1, sliced

Garlic- 2 cloves, minced

Pepper and salt- according to taste

NUTRITION INFORMATION

Fat-9 g

Fiber-0 g

Carbohydrates-0.4 g

Protein-29 g

Cholesterol-75 mg

INSTRUCTIONS:

1. Carefully line your crock pot with quality parchment paper.

2. Use pepper, salt, dill and garlic to season the salmon fillets.

3. Carefully place the seasoned fillets in the lined crock pot.

4. Place slices of lemon on the fillets.

5. Let it cook for about 2 to 3 hours on a high heat setting.

6. Slowly remove the fillets by lifting the parchment paper.

7. Serve.

SHRIMP WITH TOMATOES AND ZUCCHINI

SERVING SIZE: 1 PLATE
SERVINGS PER RECIPE: 4
CALORIES: 169
PREPARATION TIME: 1 HOURS AND 20 MINUTES

INGREDIENTS:

Olive oil- 2 tsp, extra virgin
Cherry tomatoes- 1 pint, cut
Pepper and salt- according to taste

For the shrimp:

Garlic- 1 clove, minced
Shrimp- ½ lb., large, deveined and peeled
Pepper and salt- according to taste
Olive oil- 2 tsp, extra virgin
Parsley- chopped
Lemon- 1/2

For the Zucchini:

Olive oil- 1 tsp, extra virgin
Zucchini- 2
Pepper and salt- according to taste

NUTRITION INFORMATION

Fat-2 g
Fiber-0.2 g
Carbohydrates-2 g
Protein-30 g
Cholesterol-228 mg

INSTRUCTIONS:

1. Prepare your crock pot for roasting. Choose a high temperature setting.

2. Line the crock pot with a baking sheet and layer the tomatoes on it. Make sure you grease the sheet with olive oil.

3. Add pepper and salt according to your taste and toss the tomatoes properly.

4. Let the tomatoes get roasted on a high temperature setting for about 9 to 13 minutes. When you start seeing the juices and wrinkles, stop roasting.

5. Take a large bowl to mix, the shrimp with the pepper, salt, olive oil and garlic.

6. Now, in the crock pot, add the mixture of shrimp and spices.

7. Add the cooked tomatoes with the shrimp and roast until you get cooked shrimp. This should take about 12 to 15 minutes only, depending on the size of shrimp.

8. In the meantime, you can prepare your zucchini. Add all the given ingredients for zucchini in a large pan and cook for about 1 to 3 minutes.

9. When the shrimp are ready, mix it with the zucchini.

10. Add lemon juice and garnish with parsley.

11. Serve.

SLOW COOKER SALMON WITH BASIL AND CUCUMBER

SERVING SIZE: 1 PLATE
SERVINGS PER RECIPE: 4
CALORIES: 259
PREPARATION TIME: 2 HOURS AND 13 MINUTES

INGREDIENTS:

For the marinade:

Olive oil- 1 tbsp., extra virgin

Coconut aminos- 2 tbsp.

Ginger- 1 tbsp., freshly grated

Garlic- 1 clove, crushed

Pepper flakes- 1 pinch

For the dressing:

Dijon mustard- 1 tbsp.

Olive oil- 1 tbsp., extra virgin

Honey- 1 tsp, organic

Coconut aminos- 1 tbsp., organic

Garlic- 1 clove, minced

Lemon- 1/2, juiced

Ginger- 1 ½ tbsp., freshly grated

Pepper- 1 pinch

Other ingredients:

Arugula- 3 cups

Salmon- 1 lb.

Fresh basil- ½ cup

Cucumber- 1, thinly sliced

NUTRITION INFORMATION

Fat-14 g

Fiber-1 g

Carbohydrates-7 g

Protein-24 g

Cholesterol-60 mg

INSTRUCTIONS:

1. Prepare your crock pot by layering it with a quality parchment paper.

2. Take a medium-sized bowl to combine all the marinade ingredients.

3. Season the salmon with pepper and salt after patting it thoroughly dry.

4. Coat the salmon fillets with the prepared marinade.

5. Leave for at least 4 to 8 hours.

6. Put the marinated salmon as a layer on the parchment paper in the crock pot. Cook for about 1 to 2 hours on a high temperature setting. Make sure you keep checking the salmon from time to time.

7. While the salmon is cooking, you can prepare your dressing by adding all the dressing ingredients in one bowl. Properly whisk to get a consistent mixture.

8. After cooking, let the salmon rest for about 10 minutes.

9. Serve the fish with the dressing.

SWEET AND SPICY SALMON

SERVING SIZE: 1 PLATE
SERVINGS PER RECIPE: 4
CALORIES: 408
PREPARATION TIME: 2 HOURS AND 10 MINUTES

INGREDIENTS:

Olive oil – 2 tsp

Salmon- 4 fillets

Black pepper- 1 tsp

Liquid aminos- ¼ cup

Spinach- 1 bunch

Pepper flakes- 2 tsp

Sesame oil- 2 tsp

Chili sauce and liquid aminos- for topping, use a homemade sauce

NUTRITION INFORMATION

Fat-16 g

Fiber-3 g

Carbohydrates-41 g

Protein-27 g

Cholesterol-85 mg

INSTRUCTIONS:

1. Take a large bowl to mix the liquid aminos, pepper flakes, black pepper and spinach together. Make sure you chop the spinach before mixing.

2. Use this prepared mixture as a marinade for the salmon.

3. Take a different bowl to mix the toppings with the sesame oil.

4. Now, pour a little olive oil in a crock pot and set the heat on a high temperature. Coat the salmon with the marinade thoroughly and place the pieces one by one in the crock pot.

5. Cover with the lid and cook for about 2 hours. Make sure you keep checking the fillets with a fork.

COMPLETE SEAFOOD CHILI WITH TOMATOES

SERVING SIZE: 1 BOWL
SERVINGS PER RECIPE: 4
CALORIES: 187
PREPARATION TIME: 2 HOURS AND 20 MINUTES

INGREDIENTS:

Olive oil- 1 tbsp., virgin

White onion- 1 cup, diced

Fish juice- 3 cups

Tomatoes- 14 oz., diced

Bell pepper- 1 red, diced

Jalapeno- 1, chopped

Bell pepper- 1 yellow, diced

Cumin- 1 tsp

Bell pepper- 1 green, diced

Shrimp- 1 lb., deveined

Cod loins- 2, chopped

Scallops- ½ lb., clean and dry

Clams- 6 oz., scrubbed and rinsed

Mussels- 3/4 oz., rinsed and scrubbed

Oregano- ½ tbsp.

Chili powder- 1 tbsp.

Coriander- ½ tsp

Cilantro

Salt- ¼ tsp

NUTRITION INFORMATION

Fat-2 g

Fiber-6.8 g

Carbohydrates-23 g

Protein-21 g

Cholesterol-67 mg

INSTRUCTIONS:

1. Add olive oil, bell peppers, onions, salt and jalapenos to your crock pot. Mix properly.

2. Add tomatoes, cod, clam juice and spices to the pot too. Start cooking at a low temperature for about 40 minutes.

3. After that, put the shrimp and mix properly. Let it cook covered for about 2 hours on a high temperature setting. Then, you can add the clams and mussels. Give it another 10 to 15 minutes of cooking by covering it with the lid.

4. Serve warm.

CREAMY POACHED SALMON WITH A TANGY TWIST

SERVING SIZE: 1 PLATE
SERVINGS PER RECIPE: 4
CALORIES: 211
PREPARATION TIME: 2 HOURS AND 21 MINUTES

INGREDIENTS:

Coconut milk- 1 cup

Oranges- 2, large, divided

Coco aminos- 2 tbsp.

Fish sauce- 1 tbsp., check for Whole30

Ginger- 2 tbsp., minced

Garlic- 3 cloves, minced

Salmon- 4 fillets

Lime juice- 2 tbsp.

Cilantro

NUTRITION INFORMATION

Fat-5 g

Fiber-0.9 g

Carbohydrates-5 g

Protein-30 g

Cholesterol-82 mg

INSTRUCTIONS:

1. Squeeze the orange juice into a small pan. Add the coco aminos, coconut milk, garlic, fish sauce, lime juice and ginger to the pan too. Simmer for about 3 to 6 minutes.

2. Now, transfer this mixture to the crock pot, and add the salmon fillets. Cover with the lid and cook on a high temperature heat for about 2 hours. Keep checking from time to time.

3. Use cilantro, and lime juice to garnish.

CAULIFLOWER SHRIMPS WITH CAJUN

SERVING SIZE: 1 PLATE
SERVINGS PER RECIPE: 2
CALORIES: 275
PREPARATION TIME: 2 HOURS AND 13 MINUTES

INGREDIENTS:

Cajun seasoning- 3 tbsp., look for Whole30 seasoning

Shrimp- 1 lb., large, peeled and deveined

Butter- 2 tbsp.

Salt- according to taste

Garlic- 1 clove, minced

Cauliflower- 1 bag, frozen

Salt and butter- for cauliflower

NUTRITION INFORMATION

Fat-10 g

Fiber-1 g

Carbohydrates-5 g

Protein-39 g

Cholesterol-285 mg

INSTRUCTIONS:

1. Fill enough water in the crock pot to cover the cauliflower. Add the garlic and let it steam covered on a high temperature setting. This would take about 20 to 40 minutes.

2. After that, take out the cauliflower and pulse it in your food processor. You can add a little butter and salt if required.

3. Now, use the Cajun seasoning to coat the shrimp and add them to the crock pot.

4. Add the pulsed cauliflower, water and a little salt if needed.

5. Cover the lid and let this mixture cook for about 2 to 3 hours at a high temperature setting.

6. Serve warm.

SLOW COOKER SPICY SHRIMP WITH MARINARA SAUCE

SERVING SIZE: 1 PLATE
SERVINGS PER RECIPE: 4
CALORIES: 264
PREPARATION TIME: 2 HOURS AND 32 MINUTES

INGREDIENTS:

Shrimp- 8 oz., peeled

Zucchinis- 3, spiralized

Smoked paprika- ¼ tsp

Salt- 1 pinch

Olive oil- 1 tbsp.

Tomatoes- 1 can of 15 oz., diced

Italian seasoning- 2 tsp

Garlic- 2 cloves, chopped

Red pepper- ¼ tsp, freshly crushed

Salt- according to taste

Basil

NUTRITION INFORMATION

Fat-3 g

Fiber-1 g

Carbohydrates-5 g

Protein-49 g

Cholesterol-442 mg

INSTRUCTIONS:

1. Line a large bowl with quality paper towel. Mix the zucchini with salt and put aside.

2. Now, use a pan to warm olive oil. Then, add the Italian seasoning, tomatoes and garlic. Cook for 1 minute, then, add salt and red pepper. Stir cook for another minute, then, reduce the heat and add the basil.

3. Transfer the prepared mixture of garlic and tomatoes to your crock pot, and add the shrimp. Add salt if needed.

4. Cover and let it cook for about 1 to 2 hours on a high temperature setting.

5. Now, add the zucchini and give it another 10 to 12 minutes of cooking after stirring properly.

6. Take out the shrimp and serve with basil.

WHOLE 30 CROCKPOT BEEF RECIPES

CROCK POT BEEF CURRY

SERVING SIZE: 1 BOWL
SERVINGS PER RECIPE: 8
CALORIES: 253
PREPARATION TIME: 5 HOURS AND 10 MINUTES

INGREDIENTS:

- Beef- 4 lbs., bite-size pieces, boneless
- Coconut oil- 2 tbsp.
- Onion- 1 large, chopped
- Pepper and salt- freshly ground
- Garlic- 3 cloves, minced
- Curry powder- 1 tbsp., mild
- Ginger- 3 tbsp., freshly minced
- Ground turmeric- ½ tsp
- Ground cumin- 1 tbsp.
- Coconut milk- 1 cup, not sweet
- Tomatoes- 1 can of 14 oz., diced
- Cilantro- for serving
- Chicken broth- 2 cups

NUTRITION INFORMATION

- Fat-13 g
- Fiber-1 g
- Carbohydrates-8 g
- Protein-25 g
- Cholesterol-68 mg

INSTRUCTIONS:

1. Take a large pan and warm the coconut oil. Divide the beef into multiple batches and season with pepper and salt. Then, brown the beef in batches.

2. Shift this cooked meat straight to your crockpot.

3. Mix a little meat fat with the garlic, onion, curry powder, turmeric, and cumin in a pan and cook on a medium temperature until you start getting a beautiful fragrance of garlic and onion. This won't take more than 3 to 5 minutes.

4. Shift this mixture of spices to your crock pot. Now, you can add the tomatoes, chicken broth and coconut milk.

5. Cover and give it at least 3 to 5 hours to cook properly.

6. Get rid of the excess fat from the top and serve with steamed rice.

MARINARA BEEF BALLS

SERVING SIZE: 4
SERVINGS PER RECIPE: 7 TO 8
CALORIES: 62
PREPARATION TIME: 4HOURS AND 20 MINUTES

INGREDIENTS:

For the meatballs:

Egg- 1

Ground beef- 1 ¾ lbs., lean

Sea salt- ¾ tsp

Almond flour- ¼ cup

Italian seasoning- 1 tbsp.

Garlic- ½ tsp

Parsley- 1 tbsp., fresh

Red pepper- 1 big pinch

For the sauce:

Tomatoes- 1 can, diced

Crushed tomatoes- 1 can

Onion- ½, chopped

Tomato paste- 6 oz.

Oregano leaves- 2 tbsp., fresh

Garlic- 2 tbsp., chopped

Salt- according to taste

Bay leaves- 2

NUTRITION INFORMATION

Fat-4 g

Fiber-0.1 g

Carbohydrates-0.5 g

Protein-4 g

Cholesterol-18 mg

INSTRUCTIONS:

1. To prepare the meatballs, start by mixing salt, flour, garlic, onion, red pepper and Italian seasoning together.

2. Now, take a big bowl to mix the beef with the sea salt. Add the egg and the prepared mixture of flour. Add parsley and carefully mix using your fingers. This will result in a consistent and properly bound mixture.

3. Prepare a baking sheet by lining it with parchment paper. Prepare at least 18 to 20 meatballs with the mixture. Arrange these balls carefully on the lined sheet.

4. Start broiling for about 3 to 4 minutes to get a brown color outside every ball.

5. Place these half-cooked balls in your crock pot. Make sure you remove the fat.

6. Put all the sauce ingredients in the crock pot as well. Stir slowly.

7. Cover with the lid and let the balls cook in the mixture for about 3 to 4 hours on a low heat setting.

8. Serve with veggies and garnished with fresh herbs.

ROAST BEEF WITH VEGGIES

SERVING SIZE: 1 PLATE
SERVINGS PER RECIPE: 6
CALORIES: 349
PREPARATION TIME: 8 HOURS AND 30 MINUTES

INGREDIENTS:

Pepper- ¼ tsp

Salt- ½ tsp

Beef roast- 4 lbs.

White onion- 1, small

Red potatoes- 1 ½ lbs., cut into quarter pieces

Carrots- 1 lb., peeled

Dried thyme- 1 tsp

Garlic- 1 clove, minced

Balsamic vinegar- 1/3 cup

Dried oregano- 1 tsp

Cooking oil

NUTRITION INFORMATION

Fat-9 g

Fiber-4 g

Carbohydrates-21 g

Protein-43 g

Cholesterol-111 mg

INSTRUCTIONS:

1. Season the beef roast with pepper and salt.

2. In a large pan heat some cooking oil over a medium temperature.

3. Add the meat and 1 cook it thoroughly. Put this meat into your crock pot and layer with the onion and potato pieces.

4. Add oregano, garlic, and thyme to the crock pot.

5. Pour the balsamic vinegar and top with carrots.

6. Cover with the lid and let it cook for about 7 to 8 hours on a low heat setting.

7. Carefully shred the pieces of meat and use the veggies at the time of serving.

CHILI BEEF STEW

SERVING SIZE: 1 BOWL
SERVINGS PER RECIPE: 8
CALORIES: 252
PREPARATION TIME: 6 HOURS AND 22 MINUTES

INGREDIENTS:

Ground beef- 1 lb.

Avocado oil- 1 tbsp.

Yellow onion- 1, large, diced

Bell pepper- 2, one red and one green, diced

Sweet potato- 1, small, diced after peeling

Tomato- 14 oz., diced

Chili powder- 3 tbsp.

Garlic- 1 tbsp., freshly chopped

Smoked paprika- 1 tbsp.

Crushed tomatoes- 28 oz.

Salt- 2 tsp

Cumin- 1 tbsp., ground

Chipotle chili- ½ tsp, ground

Cinnamon- ½ tsp, ground

NUTRITION INFORMATION

Fat-6 g

Fiber-4 g

Carbohydrates-27 g

Protein-20 g

Cholesterol-50 mg

INSTRUCTIONS:

1. Use a pan to warm the oil. Add the beef.

2. Stir cook to get a brown color on the meat in 3 to 5 minutes.

3. Transfer this cooked beef to your crock pot.

4. Mix together onion, peppers, sweet potato, smoked paprika, tomatoes, garlic, chili powder, cumin, chipotle, salt and cinnamon. Add this to the meat in the pot.

5. Let this cook for about 5 to 6 hours on a high heat setting.

6. Serve.

PEPPER TOMATO MUSHROOM BEEF

SERVING SIZE: 1 BOWL
SERVINGS PER RECIPE: 6
CALORIES: 233
PREPARATION TIME: 8 HOURS AND 32 MINUTES

INGREDIENTS:

Portobello mushrooms- 8 oz., sliced

Onion- 1, large, chopped

Garlic- 2 cloves

Green pepper- 1, chopped

Paprika- 2 tbsp.

Chili powder- 2 tbsp.

Ground beef- 1 lb.

Tomatoes- 2 cans, diced, undrained

Pepper and salt- according to taste

Butter- 2 tbsp.

NUTRITION INFORMATION

Fat-13 g

Fiber-6 g

Carbohydrates-13 g

Protein-19 g

Cholesterol-57 mg

INSTRUCTIONS:

1. Prepare your crock pot at a high temperature setting and add the tomatoes to it.

2. Add paprika and properly stir.

3. Use a large pan to heat the butter and cook the beef. Use a wooden spoon to properly break the meat to get a brown color.

4. Now, transfer this cooked meat to your crock pot too.

5. Also, mild cook all the vegetables and add them to the crock pot.

6. Stir the mixture in the crock pot thoroughly and add pepper and salt according to your taste.

7. Reduce the heat setting to low and cook for at least 7 to 8 hours.

8. Serve.

BEEF PASTA AND VEGETABLE SOUP

SERVING SIZE: 1 BOWL
SERVINGS PER RECIPE: 4
CALORIES: 192
PREPARATION TIME: 60 MINUTES

INGREDIENTS:

Ground beef- 1 lb., grass-fed

Coconut oil- 3 tbsp., divided

Sea salt- ½ tsp

Curry powder- 3 tsp, divided

Pepper- ¼ tsp

Carrots- 3 medium, diced

Garlic- 3 cloves, minced

Onion- 1, medium, diced

Mushrooms- 3 oz., diced

Baby kale- 2 handfuls, chopped

Tomato paste- 1 tbsp.

Pasta- 1 cup, gluten-free

Chicken broth- 2 quarts

Pepper and salt- according to taste

NUTRITION INFORMATION

Fat-3 g

Fiber-4 g

Carbohydrates-18 g

Protein-22 g

Cholesterol-46 mg

INSTRUCTIONS:

1. Add one spoon of coconut oil to your crock pot. Add the beef along with salt, curry powder and pepper. Cook to get a brown color and set aside.

2. Mix the meat juices with the veggies and sauté in a pan. Add salt and mild cook the vegetables for about 5 to 6 minutes.

3. Add the tomato paste and garlic and cook for another minute.

4. Finally, you can add the kale, chicken broth, beef, pasta and cooked vegetables to your crock pot. Let it simmer on a low heat setting for about 40 to 50 minutes. Make sure you keep checking the cooking of the pasta.

5. Add pepper and salt if required and serve.

SCALLION BEEF SOUP WITH SHIITAKE MUSHROOMS

SERVING SIZE: 1 BOWL
SERVINGS PER RECIPE: 6
CALORIES: 247
PREPARATION TIME: 2 HOURS AND 15 MINUTES

INGREDIENTS:

Carrots- 3, pieces

Beef shanks- 2 lbs., boneless cut into pieces

Tomato- 1, large, chopped

Shiitake mushrooms- 8, dry

Cinnamon stick- 1

Ginger- 4 slices

Bay leaves- 4, dry

Cumin powder- 1 tbsp.

Fennel powder- 1 ½ tbsp.

Coriander- 1 tsp, ground

Black pepper- ¼ tsp

Five spice- ¼ tsp, powder

Scallions- 1 bunch, cut and sliced

Water- 8 cups

Coconut aminos- 1/3 cup

NUTRITION INFORMATION

Fat-5 g

Fiber-6 g

Carbohydrates-29 g

Protein-22 g

Cholesterol-50 mg

INSTRUCTIONS:

1. Use a large bowl to soak the mushrooms in water.

2. Leave these pieces to soak for at least 8 hours.

3. After that, use a sharp knife to remove the stems from the mushrooms and cut into slices. You can use the mushroom water in the recipe.

4. To your crock pot add the beef shank slices along with water. Make sure that the water covers the shanks. Keep the heat on a high setting and get a boil in this mixture.

5. Now, you need to remove the shanks from the water and rinse properly by using normal temperature water.

6. Wash and prepare your crock pot to place the beef pieces again.

7. Layer with shiitake mushrooms, tomato and carrot pieces.

8. Make a teabag sized bag containing the bay leaves, cinnamon, ginger, along with all the other spices.

9. Place this packet of spices in the crock pot.

10. Cook at a high temperature setting for about 20 minutes. Then, reduce the heat setting to low and cook further for 80 to 90 minutes.

11. Make sure that the beef pieces are tender. Let it cool for at least 10 minutes. Serve.

CHIPOTLE COCOA BEEF ROAST

SERVING SIZE: 1 PLATE
SERVINGS PER RECIPE: 8
CALORIES: 212
PREPARATION TIME: 3 HOURS AND 20 MINUTES

INGREDIENTS:

Chipotle chili powder- 1 tsp
Beef roast- 2 ½ lb., grass-fed
Cumin- ¼ tsp
Cocoa powder- 1 tsp
Kosher salt- ½ tsp
Onion powder- ½ tsp

NUTRITION INFORMATION

Fat-6 g
Fiber-0.1 g
Carbohydrates-0.7 g
Protein-36 g
Cholesterol-102 mg

INSTRUCTIONS:

1. Prepare your crock pot for roasting.
2. Combine all the dry spices to create a rub for the beef roast.
3. Get rid of the unwanted fat by trimming the beef roast. Use the prepared rub to coat this roast.
4. Roast in the crock pot for 20 minutes at a high temperature setting. Then, change the temperature setting to low and let it roast for about 2 to 3 hours.
5. Ensure an internal temperature of 140 to 150 degrees.
6. Take out the meat and let it cool down for about 10 to 15 minutes.
7. Serve with potato mash.

SPINACH BEEF STEAK

SERVING SIZE: 1 STEAK
SERVINGS PER RECIPE: 2
CALORIES: 348
PREPARATION TIME: 8 HOURS

INGREDIENTS:

Beef steak- 14 oz.

Rosemary- 1 tsp, chopped

Olive oil- 1 tsp

Lemon- ¼

Sea salt- 1 tsp

Garlic- 1 clove, minced

Olive oil

Spinach- 1 cup

NUTRITION INFORMATION

Fat-13 g

Fiber-0.8 g

Carbohydrates-6.5 g

Protein-47 g

Cholesterol-137 mg

INSTRUCTIONS:

1. Prepare a marinade for the steak with the rosemary, olive oil and garlic. Rub the steak thoroughly with the marinade and leave it overnight.

2. Prepare your crock pot for the grilling process at about 500 degrees.

3. Use salt to rub the steak again and place it in the crock pot. Shift the angle after 4 minutes of cooking.

4. Add the lemon piece and cook further for about 5 to 10 minutes.

5. Follow the same process for the other side and keep grilling for 12 to 15 minutes more. Make sure that the steak is cooked through.

6. Remove and serve with a drizzle of olive oil and salt. Add the cooked spinach at the time of serving.

ABOUT THE AUTHOR

Leslie Yothers is a health and fitness enthusiast who loves teaching people about healthy ways to lose weight and live the best life they can.

Over the years, she has studied what works and what doesn't in health and fitness. She is passionate about helping others achieve great success in their diet and exercise endeavor through her books and seminars.

Her biggest satisfaction is when she finds out that she was able to help someone attain the results they've been looking for. In her free time, she loves to spend time with her 2-year-old daughter.

Made in the USA
Middletown, DE
16 June 2018